What Are You Eating?

FOOD & NUTRITION MADE SIMPLE

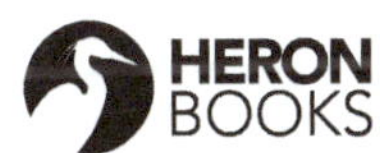

Published by
Heron Books, Inc.
20950 SW Rock Creek Road
Sheridan, OR 97378

heronbooks.com

ISBN: 978-0-89-739204-4

Printed in the USA

14 October 2020

At Heron Books, we think learning should be engaging and fun. It should be hands-on and it should allow students to move at their own pace.

For this purpose, we have created an accompanying learning guide to help the student progress through this book, lesson by lesson, with increasing confidence, interest and independence.

Get your free learning guide at *heronbooks.com/learningguides.*

For final exam, email *teacherresources@heronbooks.com.*

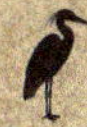

We would love to hear from you!
Email us at *feedback@heronbooks.com.*

Contents

CHAPTER 1

Food

Your body needs energy.

And it needs certain substances in order to grow.

That's what food is for. It gives the body energy to live and the things it needs to grow.

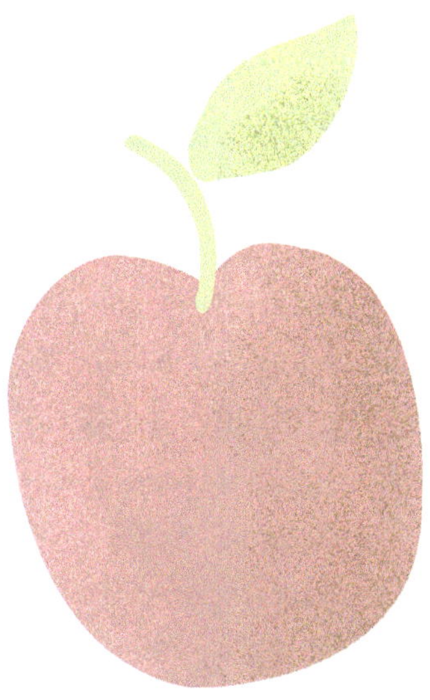

It wasn't very long ago that the most important thing about food to most people was having enough of it. There are still places in the world where this is true. If you've ever been in this situation, you know how challenging this can be!

But nowadays, in many parts of the world, most people have enough food to eat. You might think that having enough would make everybody happy about food, but actually for many of us there is so much food to choose from, it's often hard to know what foods we *should* eat.

The human body is quite an incredible thing. It will run for a surprisingly long time on many different kinds of food, even foods that aren't healthy. But sooner or later, if it doesn't have the right food, it gets tired or sick more easily. Serious illnesses can often be traced back to poor food over long periods of time.

Even common colds and the flu are easier to catch when the body isn't fed good food. You may have even experienced this in your own life, with yourself or another. People who eat well get sick less and recover faster.

It is true that youthful bodies are better at getting energy and building muscle than older bodies. They're also better at fighting off illness and repairing injuries. This is great news for young people.

On the other hand, it often leads young people to believe that what they eat isn't that important. The truth is that it does make a difference, and the eating habits you develop when you're young can influence how you eat the rest of your life.

This book was created to give you some simple information about food, to help you understand better ***what are you eating?***

The more you understand, the more you can feel confident about what foods you decide to eat.

CHAPTER 2

A Few Words to Know

Understanding the main words of a subject is always a great place to start. Here are some useful terms that will help in your study of food.

nourish:

to provide the body with those things needed for healthy life and growth. Just as good fertilizer and water nourish plants, good food and water nourish our bodies.

nutrient:

something that nourishes; any one of the substances found in food that living things *need* for life and growth.

nutrition:

food with useful nutrients in it; also, the study of the whole subject of what foods and nutrients the body needs and how they are used.

diet:

what you normally eat, your usual foods; also, a specific plan of eating to achieve some purpose, such as to become healthier or to lose weight. For instance, an athlete might eat a special diet to prepare for an activity.

digestion:

the body's process of breaking down food into tiny parts that can be absorbed into the bloodstream and used by the 30 trillion or so cells in your body.

That's 30,000,000,000 microscopic living things that need to be fed all the time!

Digestion starts in the mouth and is completed in the intestines.

Once the food gets from the intestines into your blood, it goes to the liver, which does various things to prepare it for the cells. Then the prepared food goes back into the blood where it is carried to the trillions of cells.

Just like your body overall, cells take in food and get rid of what they don't need. These waste products from the cells are returned to the bloodstream and then are carried to the intestine, bladder and lungs to be removed from the body. Some waste products even leave through the skin in the form of sweat.

These few words help you open the door to the subject of what you are eating.

Food is made of **nutrients**, which **digestion** prepares in order to **nourish** the cells. **Diet** is simply what you eat, or a special plan of eating for a particular purpose.

And this whole subject is called **nutrition**.

Next, let's talk about different kinds of nutrients.

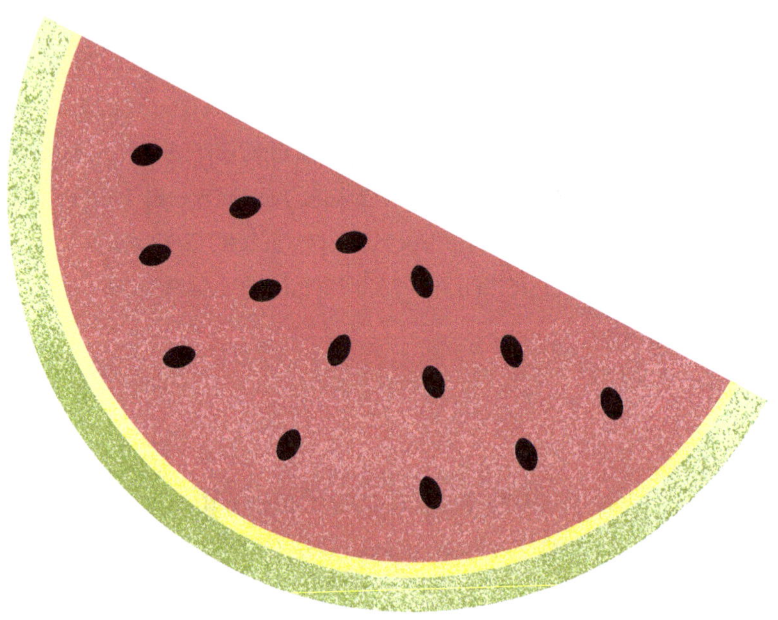

CHAPTER 3

Four Main Nutrients

With an understanding of nutrition and nutrients, you can choose the foods that will keep you healthy, strong and energetic. It's actually fairly simple, starting with four main kinds of nutrients.

CARBOHYDRATES

Carbohydrates are one of the main kinds of nutrients your body needs for energy. You may have noticed that sugar can give you a sudden feeling of energy. Sugar is a carbohydrate. But most carbohydrates come from plants, like rice, bread, beans, peas, potatoes and corn. These are called "starchy" foods because they contain a lot of starch, which is a special substance created by plants that helps them store energy.

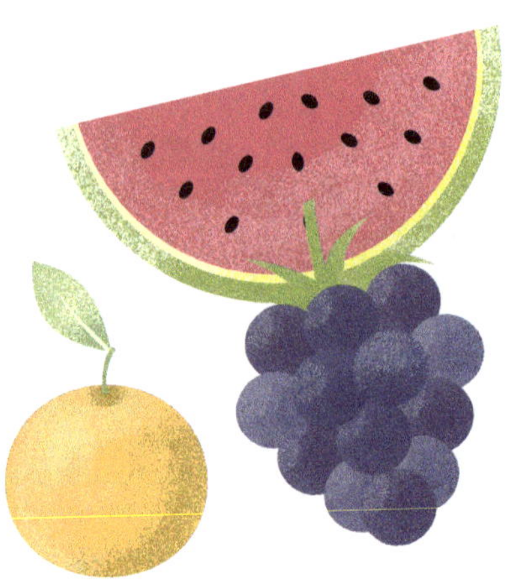

The difference between starch and sugar is that sugar gives quick energy, but often leaves you feeling tired soon afterward. Starch uses its magic to release energy into your body more gradually.

Plants and fruits all provide the body with carbohydrates. They don't all have lots of sugar or starch, but they all provide energy and other things cells need.

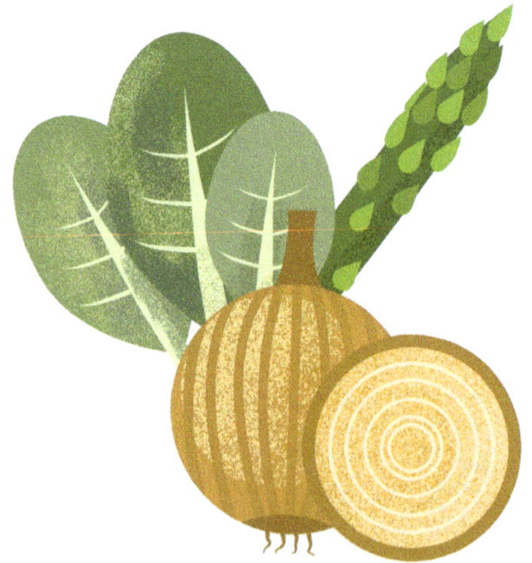

PROTEINS

Another important type of nutrient is called protein. Proteins are food substances from plants and animals that act like building blocks for cells and the body overall. Proteins are needed to make your body (muscles, bones, teeth) grow and remain strong.

Most foods contain some protein, but meats, fish, eggs, dairy products (milk, yogurt, cheese), nuts and soybeans are examples of high-protein foods.

One type of protein helps your body digest other nutrients and get longer-lasting energy from your food. Other types do different jobs inside cells. Others help your body's tissues and organs operate correctly and remain healthy and strong.

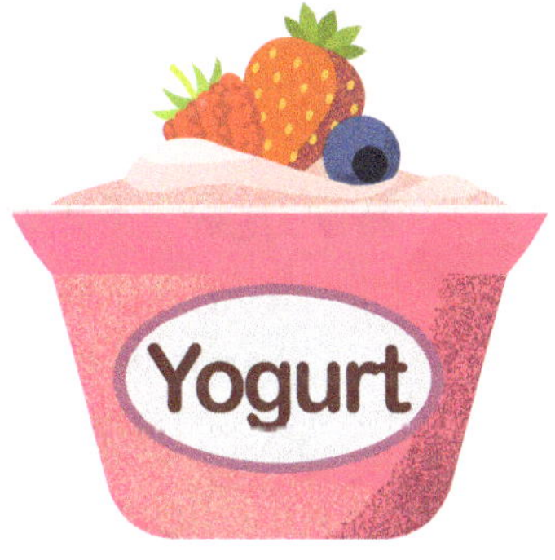

Bodies need many kinds of protein to live and grow. In fact, the breast milk a newborn gets from his or her mother contains more than 1,000 different types of protein!

FATS

Another important group of nutrients are fats. Like carbohydrates and proteins, there are many different kinds of fats. They come from both plants and animals. Some fats are basically oils while others are yellowish or whitish non-liquid substances.

Examples of fat are olive oil, vegetable oil, fat on meat, butter and mayonnaise. Many foods are high in fat, such as avocados, nuts, eggs and dairy products. Certain types of fat are not healthy for the body, like the oil many fast-food French fries are cooked in. But most fats are very important to the body.

A few of the jobs of fats are to store energy, to make strong cells, and to protect organs. Certain vitamins the body needs to live can only be absorbed by fats. Fats even assist the brain to function properly.

WATER

We usually don't think of water as a food or nutrient, but our bodies are mostly water (about 60%!) and we need a lot of it to keep from drying up. Even though much of our food (except oils/fats) contains a lot of water, it doesn't give us the amount we need. There are two reasons our bodies need plenty of water:

1. Getting food to the cells.

   The nutrients we eat are carried to the cells through the blood, and blood is mainly made of water. To live, our cells need nutrients. To get those nutrients, the blood needs water.

2. Taking wastes from the cells.

   Wastes and harmful substances are taken away from the cells by the blood, and many of them are taken away from the body in urine. If you don't drink enough water, the organs that make, store and carry off urine can even get infected. They need to get rid of those wastes!

In addition to solid foods containing carbohydrates, proteins and fats, the human body needs plenty of liquids (water, milk, juices, etc.) every day.

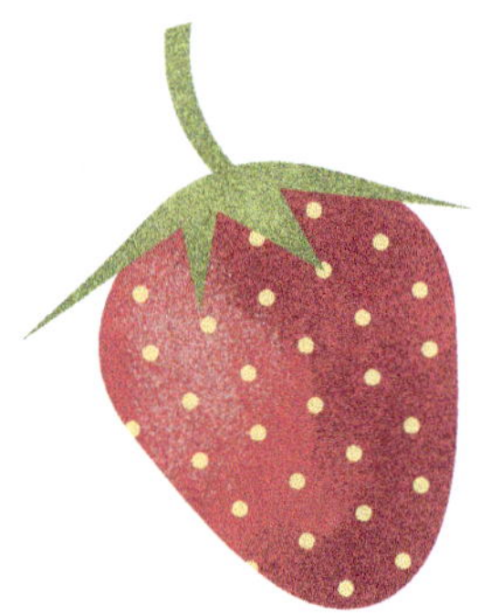

CHAPTER 4

Vitamins, Minerals and Fiber

In addition to the main nutrients discussed in Chapter 3, our bodies need a few more things to live and grow.

VITAMINS

Vitamins are very small nutrients that mostly come from plants and animals. They serve many vital functions throughout your body.

You have probably heard of different vitamins by their names, like Vitamin A, which helps your eyes and supports cell growth, or Vitamin C, which helps your body fight illness and heal wounds. Vitamin D, which helps build strong bones, comes from very few foods such as salmon and tuna or egg yolks. But your body can make vitamin D if it gets enough sunlight!

MINERALS

Minerals are substances like salt or iron. They are obtained from plants, animals and water. Like vitamins, minerals are tiny nutrients that perform many important functions in the body.

Some minerals you may have heard of are calcium, which helps build bones and keep your heart beating, or magnesium, which helps your muscles and nerves work properly.

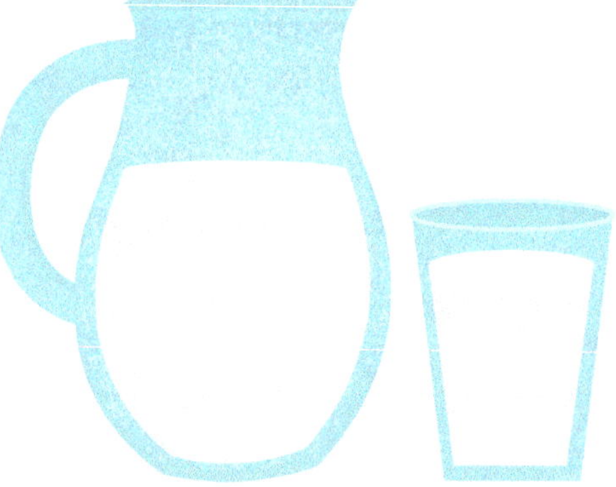

WHAT VITAMINS AND MINERALS DO

Truthfully, there are so many things that vitamins and minerals are needed for in the body, it's easier to ask, "What DON'T vitamins and minerals do?"

If you were to study all the millions of small and large functions throughout a human body, you would find vitamins and minerals playing important roles in ensuring those functions are successful. Certain vitamins and minerals are needed in only very small amounts, but that doesn't make their jobs any less important.

Sometimes a person doesn't get all the vitamins and minerals they need from the foods they eat. This is especially true nowadays when people often eat less fresh and natural food than they did in the past. Many people take "supplements" (specially prepared pills or liquids with extra vitamins) to make up for the lower quality of food.

Vitamins and minerals help regulate the change of food to energy in the body. They also help defend the body against damaging substances, whether those substances are produced in the body (such as wastes), enter through the digestive system (such as alcohol) or through the skin (such as radiation from the sun or things like x-ray machines).

They often work together, and they also work in partnership with special proteins that can't do their jobs without certain vitamins and minerals.

FIBER

Fiber is tiny "strings" in some foods that don't digest, so they just pass on through your body. Fiber is a type of carbohydrate, but because it is not absorbed by the body, it is not really a nutrient.

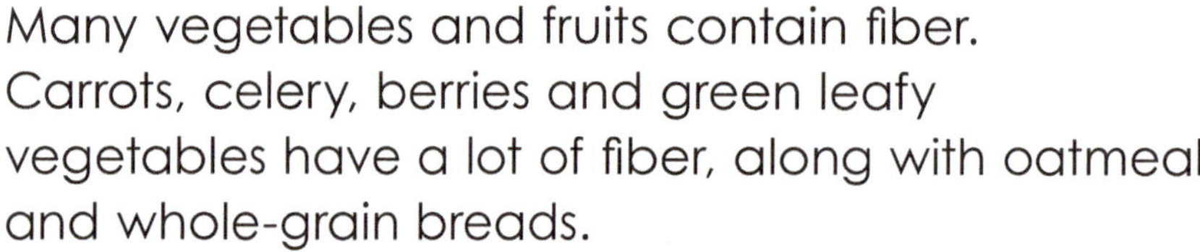

Many vegetables and fruits contain fiber. Carrots, celery, berries and green leafy vegetables have a lot of fiber, along with oatmeal and whole-grain breads.

Fiber helps the body do its work of moving food through the stomach and intestines so it gets digested and is easy to expel when you go to the bathroom. Some kinds of fiber are even important in keeping fat deposits from building up in your blood vessels (which can put extra strain on your heart).

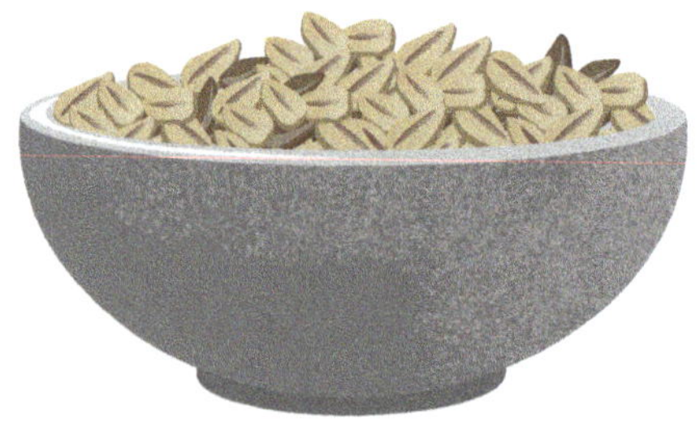

Along with the four main nutrients of carbohydrates, proteins, fats and water, vitamins, minerals and fiber are necessary for a healthy body.

So, what are you eating? You're eating all those things. But how much of each do you need for the best health?

To answer that you need to know more about what different kinds of foods do.

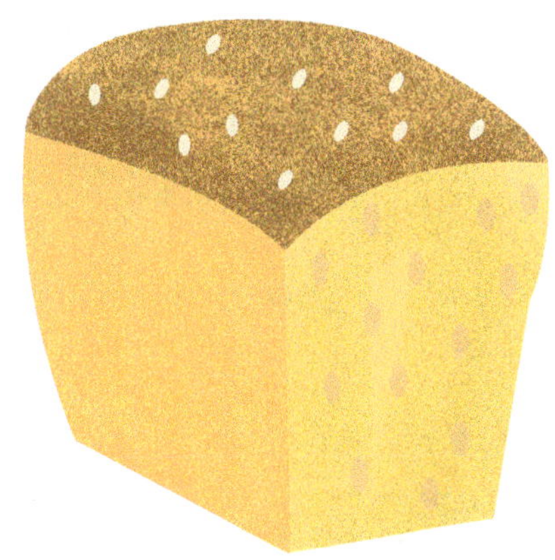

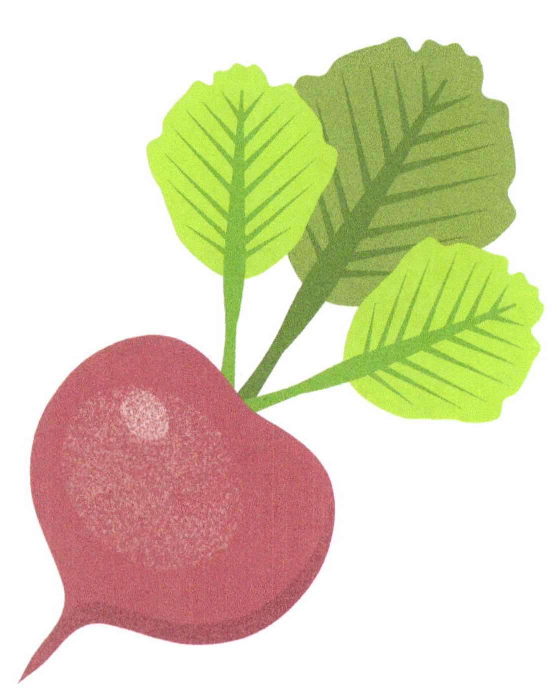

CHAPTER 5

Food Groups

Food can be grouped in different ways. Some nutritionists and countries break food down into four, five or even six different food groups. To keep things simple, we're going to focus on just three groups.

GROUP 1: CARBOHYDRATES.

This group has two parts—non-starchy carbohydrates and starchy carbohydrates. This is because these provide nutrients in different quantities.

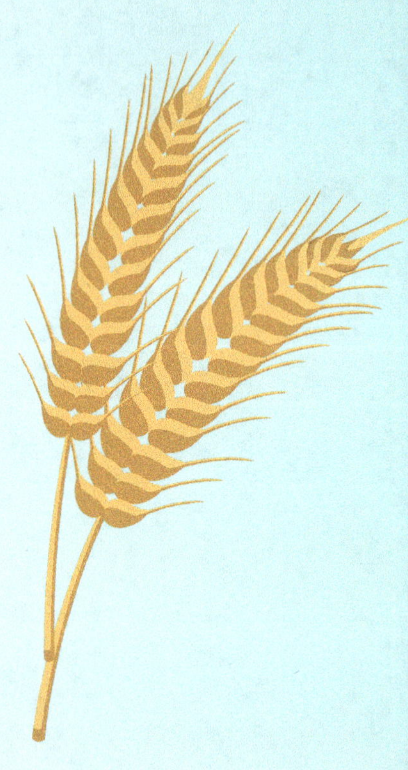

GROUP 2: PROTEINS.

Most foods contain some protein, but the foods we're putting in this grouping are ones that are particularly high in protein.

GROUP 3: REFINED SWEETS AND UNHEALTHY FATS

Refined[1] sweets are foods with refined sugar, which is when sugar cane or sugar beets go through a process that takes everything away except the sugar.

Some refined sweets are made with high-fructose corn syrup. Fructose is the natural sugar in

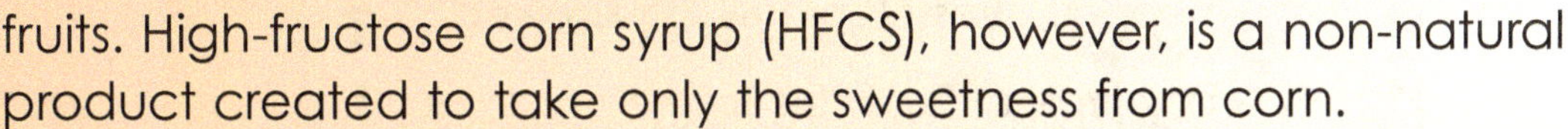

fruits. High-fructose corn syrup (HFCS), however, is a non-natural product created to take only the sweetness from corn.

When nature's foods have been refined this way, the sugar that results is way over-balanced, as the other nutrients that were naturally there have been stripped away.

Unhealthy fats are vegetable oils that have been changed so they don't break down in cooking and last longer. These are commonly called "trans fats" or "partially hydrogenated oil." There are complicated chemical reasons for these names, but the important thing to know is how they affect your body. They increase the chances for heart attack, stroke[2] and diabetes[3]. There is no known nutritional value for these fats.

---

1 **refined**: when you refine something, you change it, usually to make it more pure by taking out unwanted parts. For example, if you have rock with copper in it, you can refine the substance so that you only have copper.

2 **stroke**: a serious injury to the brain when a blood vessel clogs or bursts.

3 **diabetes**: a disease that affects how the amount of sugar is controlled in the body.

The following table gives examples of foods in each of these groups. It also shows the nutrients your body gets from each.

Food Groups

FOOD GROUP	FOODS	THE MAIN THINGS YOUR BODY GETS FROM THE FOOD
Group 1a Non-starchy carbohydrates	leafy vegetables, such as lettuce, kale, spinach, cabbage, arugula vegetables such as carrots, broccoli, radishes, celery, zucchini, bell peppers, Brussel sprouts, cauliflower any type of fruit, plus juice	carbohydrates, vitamins, minerals, fiber
Group 1b Starchy carbohydrates	any type of bread, crackers, tortillas, pasta, rice, oatmeal, potatoes, corn	carbohydrates, minerals, some fiber, some vitamins
Group 2 Proteins	beef, pork, chicken, turkey, fish, eggs, milk, yogurt, cheese, cottage cheese, nuts and nut butters beans and soybean products (which are carbohydrates but included here because they are high-protein vegetables)	protein, vitamins, minerals
Group 3 Refined sweets and unhealthy fats	table sugar, jam and jelly, syrup, refined honey, candy, soda margarine and many packaged foods and fried foods—especially fried fast food—that use partially hydrogenated oils	very few, if any, nutrients

WHAT FOODS ARE BEST?

While there is general agreement that Group 3 foods, especially in large amounts, are unhealthy, there is less agreement on what combination of food groups works best for everyone. A person's age, size and activity level will influence the needs of the body. Some people do better emphasizing more proteins over carbohydrates, while others work best with those reversed.

To help you make decisions about your diet, the next table explains what can happen if a person eats too much or too little of any food group.

FOOD GROUP	WHAT CAN HAPPEN WHEN YOU EAT TOO MUCH FOR TOO LONG	WHAT CAN HAPPEN WHEN YOU EAT TOO LITTLE FOR TOO LONG	COMMENTS
Group 1a Non-starchy carbohydrates (fruits and vegetables)	diarrhea	constipation[4]; general poor health. In extreme cases, heart disease and blood circulation problems	Fruits and non-starchy vegetables provide some of every kind of food nutrient you need, including fiber and vitamins.
Group 1b Starchy carbohydrates (bread, pasta, rice, etc.)	weight gain; could develop heart and blood circulation problems	lack of quick energy, loss of weight	The main use of starchy vegetables is fuel for quick energy.

4 **constipation**: when a person's stools (poop) don't come out easily or often enough. Passing stools out of the body is called bowel movement. Most people have at least one bowel movement a day though some people have only a few a week. When the stools are too hard and don't pass out of the body easily, it can be very uncomfortable.

FOOD GROUP	WHAT CAN HAPPEN WHEN YOU EAT TOO MUCH FOR TOO LONG	WHAT CAN HAPPEN WHEN YOU EAT TOO LITTLE FOR TOO LONG	COMMENTS
Group 2 Proteins	stomach aches, feeling tired, headaches, harm to vital organs like heart, kidney, liver	lack of growth, low resistance to disease, lack of longer-lasting energy, general poor health	Dairy products are proteins that provide our most concentrated sources of calcium, a mineral needed to grow strong bones and teeth.
Group 3 Refined sweets and unhealthy fats	weight gain, heart and circulation problems, low energy, tooth decay, increased risk of diabetes	Nothing bad can happen from avoiding these. Removing them results in better health.	

CHAPTER 6

Energy and Food

A body needs energy to live, and the more you want to do, the more energy you need. So, let's talk about food and the energy it provides.

Something all foods have in common is that they make it possible for your body to grow and to move. To move at all, you need energy—and all foods have some energy in them.

Think about it this way: Hunger is how your body tells you that it has used up the energy it got from food and needs more. If you eat a very big meal, you won't be hungry for a while. This is because more food equals more energy, and so you go longer before you feel hungry. If, on the other hand, you have a very small meal, you'll soon be hungry again. This is because you consumed less energy and your body used it all up faster.

Now, what happens if you constantly consume more energy than your body uses? Your body saves this extra energy in the form of fat. This is a useful trick of the body. It makes sure to save some energy for when you need it. Of course, it is possible to have too much fat, which is when the body has stored more energy as fat than you can easily use up.

The amount of energy in food can be measured. The unit we use to measure the energy in food is called a **calorie**. For example, a carrot can have 40 calories, a piece of chicken breast can have 230, a small bag of chips can have 240 calories, and a bacon cheeseburger can have up to 920 calories! It would take you twenty-three carrots to get the same amount of energy as one cheeseburger!

You may be wondering how many calories you need to eat in a day—how much energy your body needs. This depends on things like how old you are, how big you are, and how much physical activity you are doing in a normal day.

To calculate what this number is for you, you can search "calorie calculator" online. A calorie calculator asks for some information, and then gives a number. For example, it will tell you that a 15-year-old male, who is 5 feet 6 inches tall, weighs 120 lbs., and plays soccer every day, would need to eat around 2,300 calories to maintain his weight. If he ate less than that, he would soon start losing weight because the body would have to use up all its stored energy. If he ate more than that, he would begin to gain weight as the body stored up the extra energy in fat.

Calorie calculators can be used to figure out how many calories you should eat to maintain your normal growth. They can't say exactly, of course, but they will give you a good idea.

Also, if a person is trying to lose weight or gain weight, they can use a calorie calculator and then watch carefully what they eat, targeting more calories to gain weight or fewer calories to lose weight.

Of course, remaining healthy and strong is not just about how many calories you take in every day. Usually your natural hunger will take care of that. It's more about eating the calories (food) that will nourish your body and help you feel, move and think better.

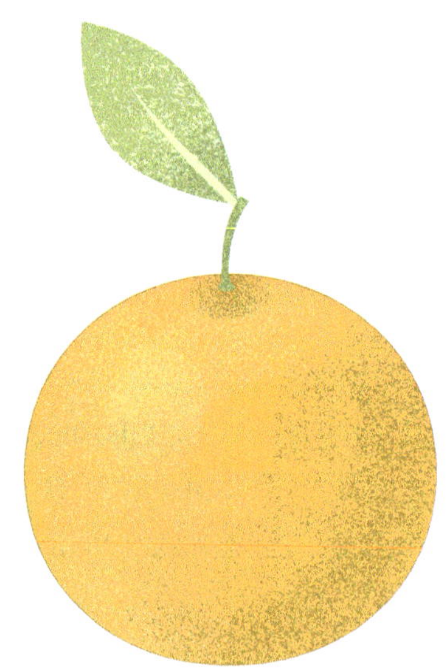

CHAPTER 7

Do I Really Want To Eat That?

If a food is highly nutritious, it tends to spoil more easily than a food that is not so nutritious. The reason for this is that if a food is good for you, then the smaller life forms like bacteria and fungus like it too. It's unwanted bacteria and fungus that spoil food.

REFINED FOOD

The food industry[5] has the problem of figuring out how to keep food products from spoiling so that they can be stored for a long time. Of course, refrigerators and canned foods are two ways to prevent or slow spoilage. The food industry has also developed other methods, such as refining foods by removing certain nutrients. They also refine food by adding certain ingredients that make it taste better, even if those ingredients aren't good for you.

Foods that are rich in carbohydrate naturally have some fiber, some vitamins and minerals, and sometimes some protein or oil. When the food is refined, much of this is lost. For example, when wheat and rice are refined, protein, fiber, calcium, iron and certain vitamins are greatly reduced.

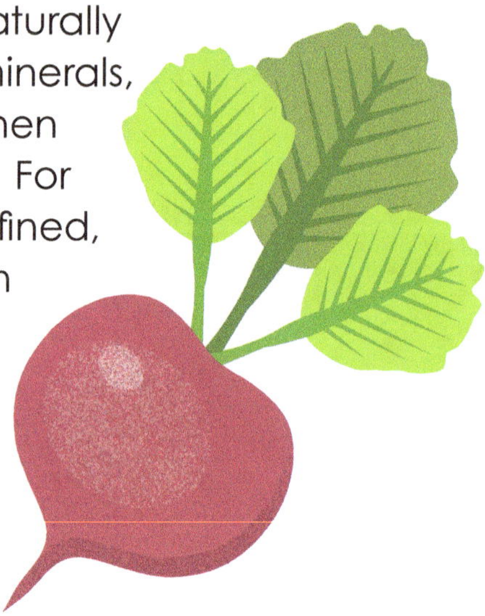

5 **food industry:** The food industry includes all the activities and businesses involved in supplying food such as farming, storage, distributing, processing, preserving, selling, etc.

When sugar is refined from the juice of sugar beets and sugar cane, a number of things are removed—calcium, iron, vitamins, and a great deal of fiber.

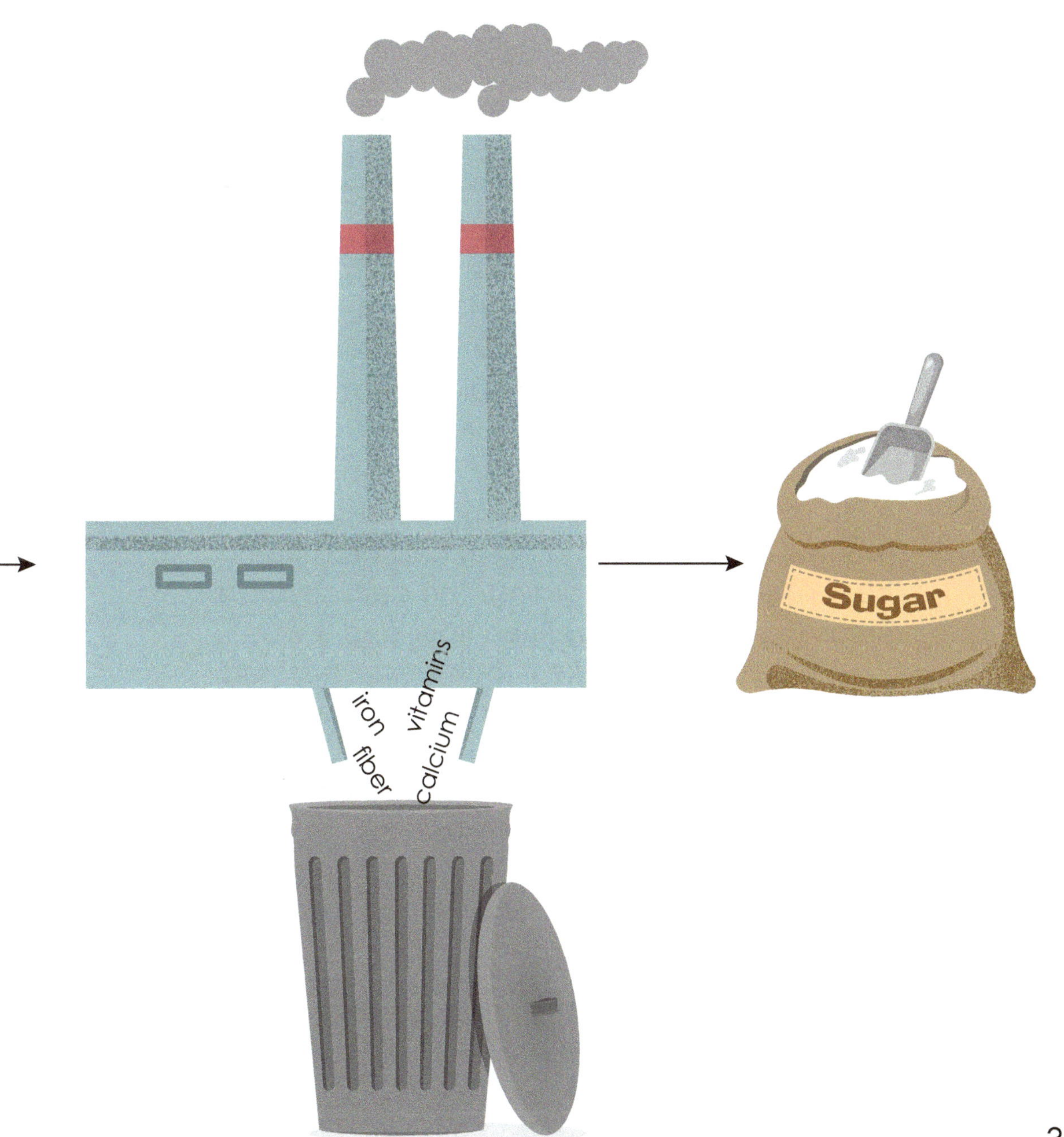

Refined Flour

Products made from refined wheat flour are a common source of refined carbohydrates.

Most of a wheat grain is carbohydrate (mainly starch), but each grain is also covered with an outer fiber layer called **bran**, and the part from which a new wheat plant might grow, called the **wheat germ**. Although the wheat germ is a small part of the wheat grain, it is rich in nutrients including protein and oil. Until the 1800s, bread was normally made from whole wheat grains ground into whole wheat flour.

In the mid-1800s, a flour-making process was invented to separate the germ and bran from the wheat (and other grains). The carbohydrate remaining was called **refined flour** and it was often bleached to make it look whiter. It stored quite well and the insects left it alone, but it didn't have much nutritional value because it was mostly starch stripped of fiber and other nutrients—that's why the insects weren't interested in it.

Today refined flour is used to make all kinds of pastas, crackers, cookies and breads. It is usually called "enriched" flour on ingredient labels because a few vitamins have been added back in. Lacking the bran and fiber which would make your stomach work for nutrients and give you energy over a longer period of time, you can experience a quick rush of energy and then a letdown. Interestingly, the wheat germ (the most nutritious part of the wheat grain) and wheat bran (a source of fiber) are now sold separately.

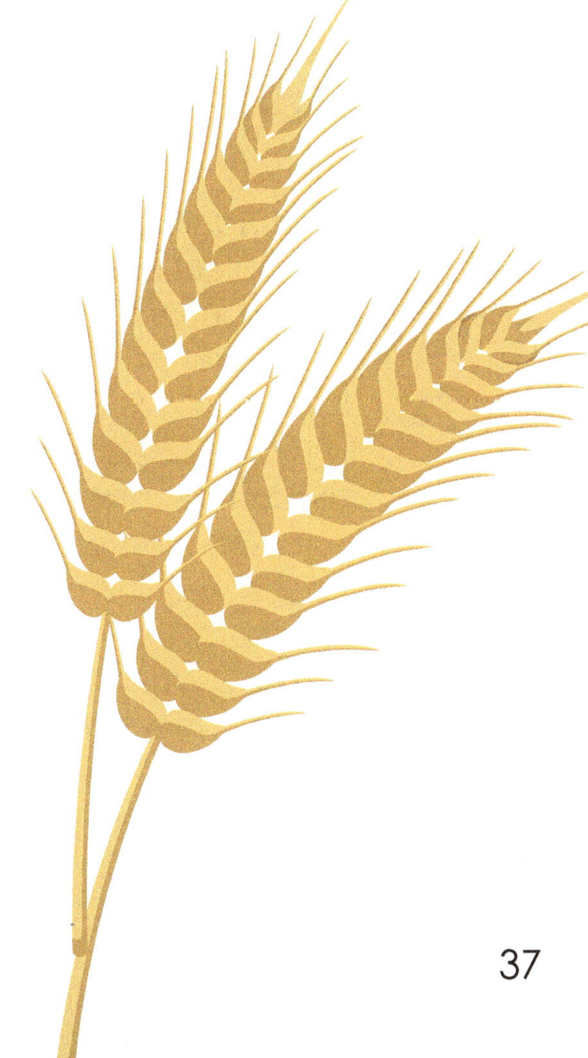

PROCESSED FOODS

Processed food is food prepared or changed by special treatment, for example adding chemicals to give it texture, color, flavor, body or to give it longer storage life on the shelf.

Some processed foods have more additives than others. Sometimes there are so many ingredients

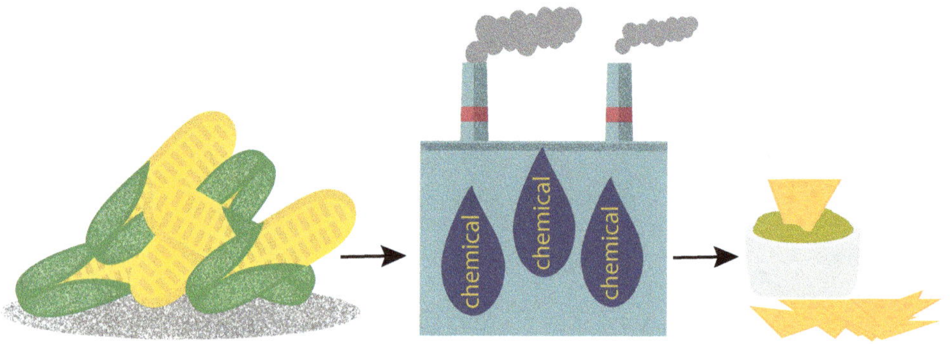

and additives that it is hard to tell what the main ingredient is. And unless you are a chemist, you can't understand what many of the ingredients even are!

Highly processed foods have become a major part of the diet of many people today. Unless you prepare most of your meals from basic ingredients (not mixes), it is hard to avoid processed foods and additives. Just about any packaged food you pick up has some chemicals added, and the ones for making mixes and sauces have the most.

Refined sugar is also an ingredient in a tremendous number of packaged foods, including just about every kind of dry cereal, not to mention protein bars, granola, yogurt, baked beans, sauces and sports drinks.

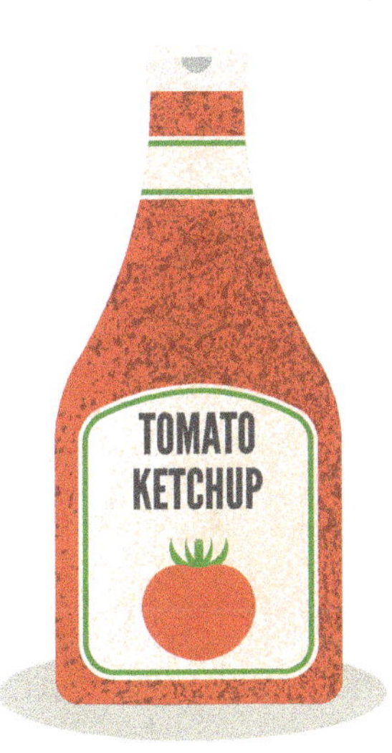

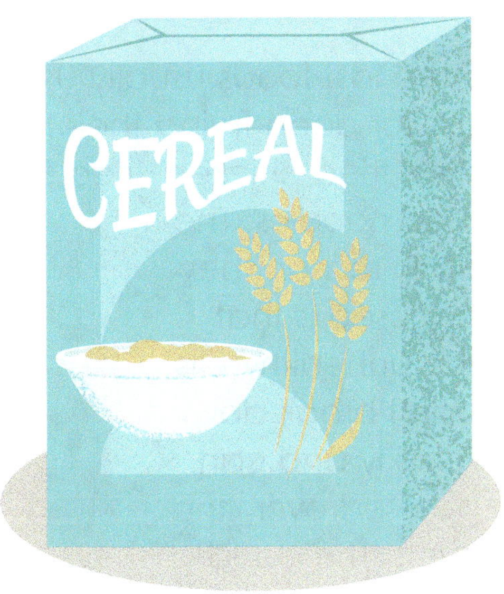

tomatoes
vinegar
sugar
salt
spice
natural flavoring

whole grain oat flour
sugar
corn flour
whole wheat flour
rice flour
salt
calcium carbonate
disodium phosphate
reduced iron
niacinamide
zinc oxide
BHT (a preservative)
yellow 5
yellow 6
thiamin mononitrate
pyridoxine hydrochloride
riboflavin
folic acid

JUNK FOODS

Junk foods are foods that are full of refined ingredients like carbohydrates, fats and sugar, but have few other nutrients. They often have many chemicals added. They are called junk foods because they aren't balanced nutritionally, and eating lots of them is hard on the body.

Here are a few examples of junk food:

1. Fried fast foods usually use unhealthy oils for deep-frying their French fries, fried chicken, fried fish and fried noodles. The main reason they are used is that the unhealthy oils don't break down quickly and can be used over and over. (The good news is that some states and countries are working to limit or eliminate this use in restaurants.)

   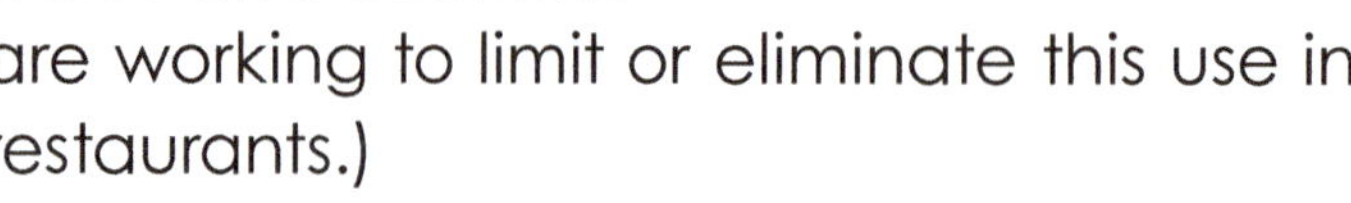

   Potato chips are mostly starch. Corn chips are similar, but may have more nutrients and fiber.

2. Candy and soft drinks are full of sugar and/or high fructose corn syrup (HFCS), another type of refined sugar.

3. Some foods and drinks contain artificial sweeteners instead of sugar. These chemicals are not nutrients because the body doesn't digest them. They are known to cause some people physical problems. Some common ones are aspartame, sucralose and saccharin with brand names like NutraSweet®, Equal®, Sweet'N Low® and Splenda®. Though all approved for use in the U.S., some countries don't allow some of them in food.

Many packaged desserts and snacks are loaded with refined sugar, refined flour and trans fats and have many chemicals added to keep them from spoiling.

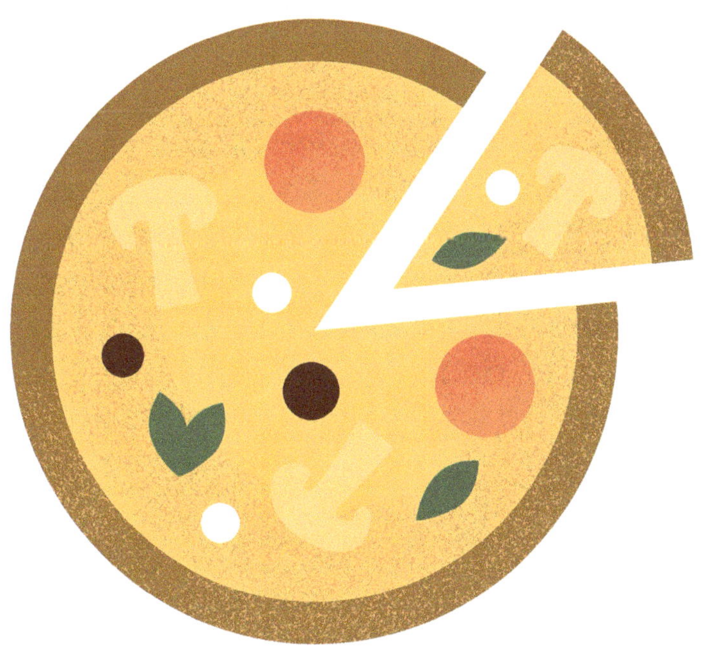

EFFECTS ON THE BODY

While foods that have been refined and highly processed are food, they are not balanced because most or all of their natural nutrients and fiber have been taken away—not to mention the chemicals that have been added. It's not healthy to eat a lot of these refined foods for long periods of time because they don't give the body all the nutrients it needs to function. Eating a diet heavy in refined and processed foods over time can cause weight gain and other health problems.

Although some people are tempted to eat a lot of high-sugar foods, it is harder on your body than you might think. Substituting fruit for refined sugar gives you fiber, vitamins and minerals to balance the sugar. Raw (not refined) honey is a better choice because it also contains some vitamins and minerals.

The human body needs good nutrition to stay healthy, grow strong bones, build muscle, and maintain energy for activities throughout the day. While it may be able to handle refined, processed, and junk food in moderation, when looking at your longer-term diet you might want to ask yourself, "Do I really want to eat that?"

CHAPTER 8

So What Should You Eat?

The first thing to know as you begin learning about what you, personally, should eat, is that not all nutritionists agree on what a correct diet is.

The science of nutrition is always changing as scientists, nutritionists and health professionals continue to learn. Some things that were recommended twenty or thirty years ago are not recommended any more. And some things that were not recommended at an earlier time are now commonly considered okay.

Additionally, each body is somewhat different, and one kind of diet may not be right for everyone. The best diet for a person depends on many things, such as the kind of body they have, how healthy they are, how active they are, their age, and so on.

There are some things that almost all nutritionists and health professionals agree on, such as that eating a lot of vegetables is good. However, some think that you should eat a lot of carbohydrate and only a little fat, while others think you should eat a lot of protein and fat but not much carbohydrate.

Even though nutritionists have different ideas about how much of your nutrition should come from carbohydrates, protein and fat, all would agree that the amount of *refined and processed foods* in the modern diet, such as white bread, snack foods, chips, pastries, sodas and sweetened breakfast cereals, is much too high.

EATING FOR GROWING BODIES

A growing body has needs that are different from those of an adult. The fact that you are building muscle, bones and teeth should be a factor when choosing foods. Even growing bodies are different in terms of how food should be balanced for each person, but here are two general suggestions that you can consider in figuring out what you should eat.

- Eat a variety of foods from the first two food groups (carbohydrates and protein) every day because different foods in each group provide different nutrients.

- Don't eat too much or too little from these food groups. Eat in moderation.

But let's take a look more closely.

Carbohydrates

- Normally, a fair amount of your food should come from carbohydrates (fruits, vegetables, whole grains).

- Fruits and vegetables hold their nutrition best if they are fresh or are fresh frozen, and then eaten raw or without a lot of cooking. They lose some of their nutrition when they are cooked, get old or when they are canned.

- It's best to avoid refined carbohydrates, including sweets, when you can. Eating lots of these foods, which can cause weight gain in the teen years, is linked to body troubles later in life, including obesity, heart and circulatory problems, and other serious, life-shortening conditions.

- If you can't avoid these foods, the best time to eat them is when you are exercising hard. Right before, during and immediately after exercising, healthy bodies can use carbohydrates and sugar for energy well. At other times your body might turn it into fat instead. However, even when exercising, fruit is a better source of sugar.

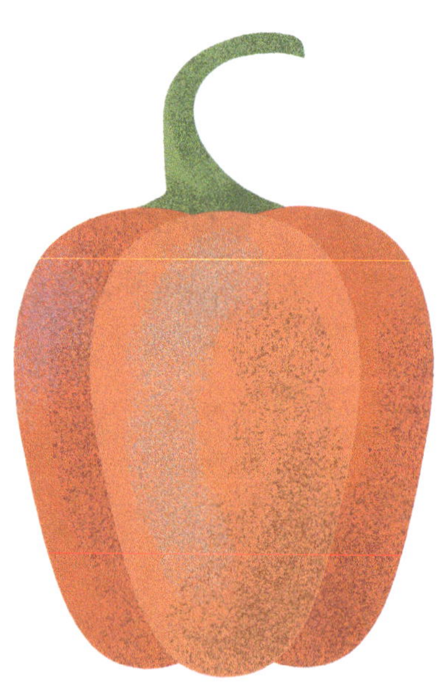

Protein

- Be sure to get some protein each day because your body needs it for growth and tissue repair.

- In addition to providing protein, dairy (milk, yogurt, cheese) and soybean products are good sources of the mineral, calcium. Calcium is needed to grow strong teeth and bones (especially important if you are involved in any athletic activity).

- Proteins from animal foods (for example, fish, meat, eggs, milk) are called "complete" proteins, which means they contain everything that you need from protein.

- You can also get protein by eating only plant foods, but plant proteins are "incomplete." To make these a complete protein, you can combine different plant foods to "get all the parts." Beans, peas, peanuts, and soybeans belong to a class of plants called legumes. You can usually make a plant food a complete protein by combining it with legumes. For instance, rice and beans make a complete protein. So does peanut butter on whole wheat toast.

- Research has shown that another option for meeting protein needs with a plant-based diet is to eat a *variety* of plant protein sources throughout the day.

Fat

- Fat is nearly always present in the protein food you eat. But if you add fat to your diet, some healthy foods to try would be extra-virgin olive oil, nuts, olives, avocados and fish.

Fiber

- Most people need more fiber in their diet than they get. If you eat enough *unrefined* carbohydrate, then you will also get enough fiber and won't have to worry about this one. This means eating whole grains, vegetables and fresh fruit such as apples, bananas, oranges, pears and berries.

When you look at it, there are many choices for healthy, nutritious food!

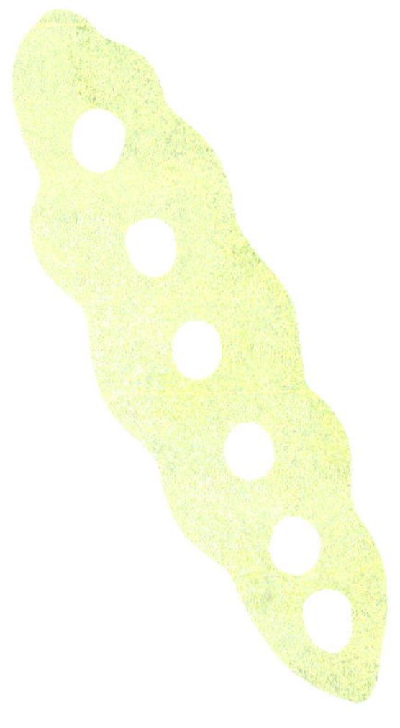

CHAPTER 9

Meal Ideas

Once you have some basic knowledge of nutrition, it can be fun and challenging to create a meal plan for yourself. Some tips and ideas are given here.

BREAKFAST

Don't skip breakfast—it helps you feel alert and energetic throughout the day.

Many nutritionists would say that a good breakfast for a growing young person might include a carbohydrate and a protein. The carbohydrate gives quick energy to get you started, and the protein helps keep you fueled and full until the next meal.

Nutritionists would also agree that a good breakfast would not include sugar and refined/processed foods.

Carbohydrate Sources

- fresh fruit or unstrained fruit juice
- whole grain cereal (such as oatmeal, granola, whole wheat, barley)
- vegetables (such as included in an omelet or quiche)
- whole grain bread (such as whole wheat or multi-grained)

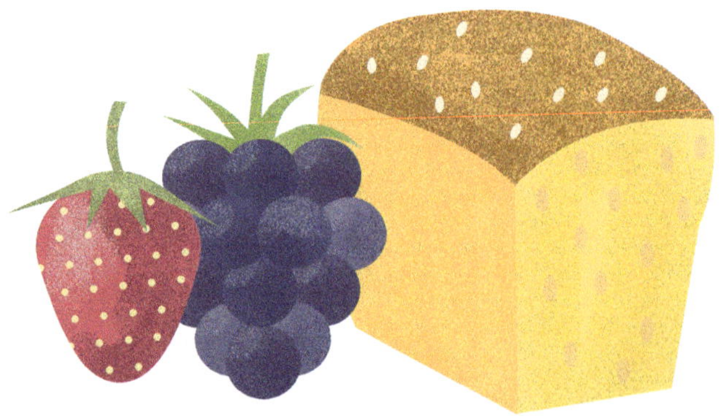

Protein Sources

- eggs
- low-sugar yogurt
- meat
- cheese
- milk
- fish

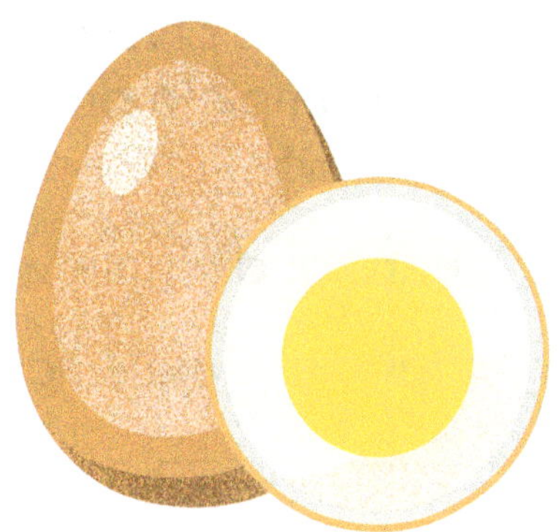

LUNCH AND DINNER

- Salads with raw vegetables in them (tomatoes, radishes, cucumbers, sprouts, bell peppers, etc.), served plain, with salad dressing or perhaps with lemon juice and olive oil. Such salads provide healthy carbohydrates, fiber, vitamins, minerals and fat (in the salad dressing oil).

- At least one other vegetable (raw or lightly cooked) with each meal. Examples: carrots, spinach, potatoes, turnips, asparagus, artichokes, beans, peas, broccoli, cabbage, etc. Some of these could be in soups. These vegetables provide carbohydrates, fiber, vitamins and minerals. When cooked in oil or butter, or with butter added, these also provide fat.

- A protein source with each meal. Any animal protein such as chicken, fish, eggs, cheese, beef, etc., are complete proteins. Here are some good complete plant proteins:
    - beans and whole wheat bread
    - peas and whole rice
    - beans and corn
    - peanuts and sunflower seeds
    - beans and whole rice
    - soybean curd (tofu) and grains
    - nuts and vegetables

SNACKS

- Have healthy snacks if you get hungry or low on energy between meals.
- For quick energy, eat fruit. On an empty stomach it takes about 20 minutes for the sugar from the fruit to get to the small intestine and to be absorbed into the bloodstream.

Snack Ideas

- whole grain bagel with peanut or other nut butter
- raw vegetables with yogurt dip
- hardboiled egg
- protein smoothie

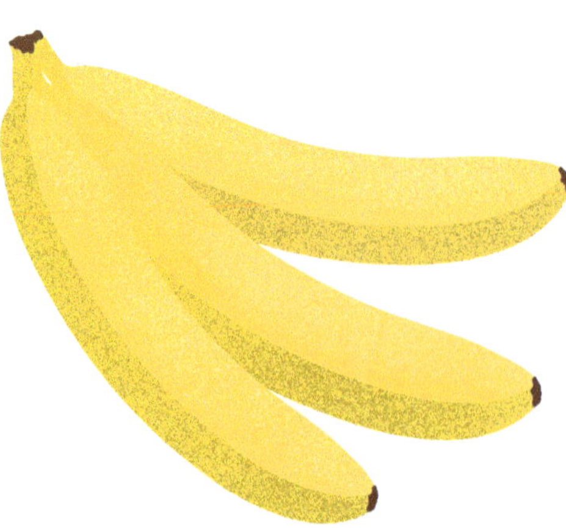

- hummus or nut butter with whole grain cracker
- cheese sticks
- popcorn
- handful of nuts
- whole grain cereal with milk

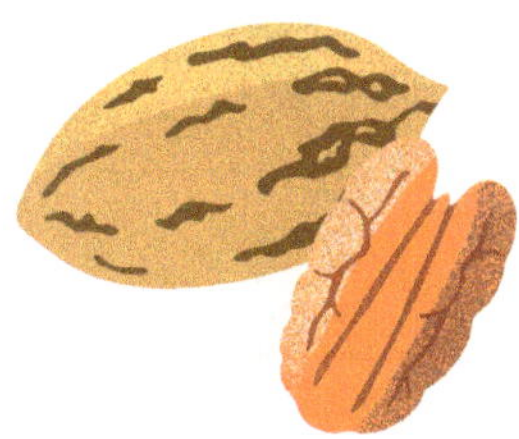

Again we can see how many choices for healthy food there are!

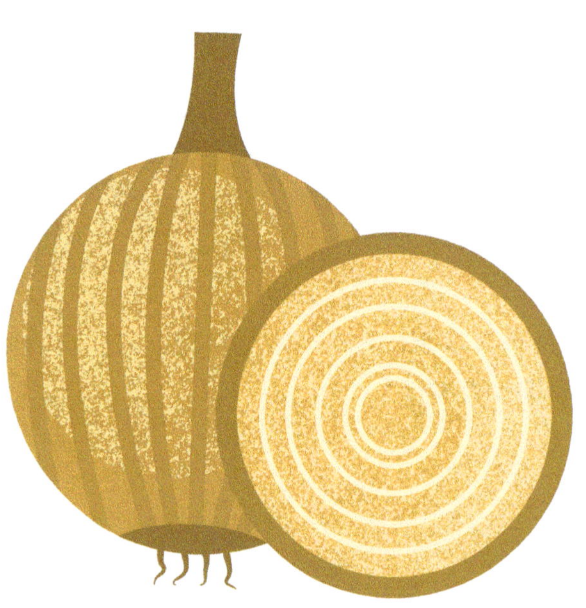

CHAPTER 10

So Much More To Know

You've learned quite a bit about food and nutrition. Here are a few more things you might find interesting.

If you look at cultures where people tend to have good health and a longer life, you'll find that they generally eat an unrefined carbohydrate/low-fat diet, which includes a moderate amount of protein.

For instance, Japanese and Southeast Asians eat a diet abundant in rice and vegetables with only small amounts of protein, and they suffer little heart disease compared to people in the Western countries.

On the other hand, there may be other nutritional reasons for long life, and simpler ones at that. For instance, research on animals has shown that simply *eating less* (provided you are getting all the nutrients you need) might be a reason for a longer life, rather than specifically *what* you eat. When rats and monkeys were kept on a diet that was 10–20% less than they normally liked to eat, they didn't age as fast and lived longer.

So while it is true that many Asians eat an unrefined carbohydrate/low-fat/moderate protein diet, they also tend to eat *less* food. In many Western countries, large portion sizes are common (such as the "super-sized" meals that fast-food restaurants promote). If you have grown up in the United States, you might notice when traveling to other countries that the plates are smaller there! The message from this might be to make a habit of eating less and to leave the table before being totally full. That way our bodies have to use the food we eat more efficiently.

And here's another interesting thing people have noticed about food and nutrition: if you tried something you don't normally eat and it didn't taste good, it might not be the food that is to blame, or even you! Food tastes best when it is freshest and well prepared. Sure, you won't like every kind of food. But keep in mind that most food tastes good because your body knows it is healthy! If it is fresh and well prepared, it almost always tastes good.

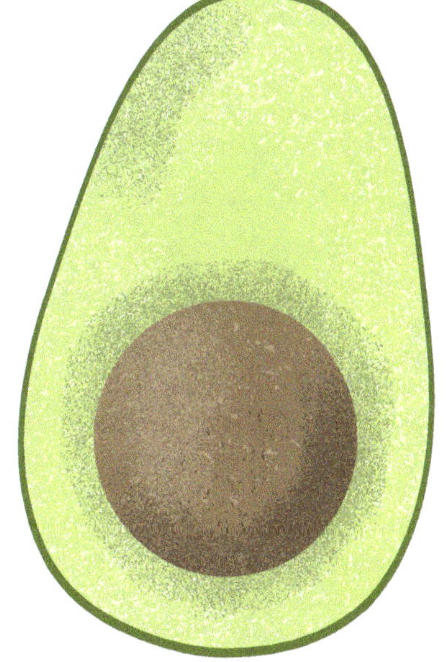

So, yes, there are many interesting things to learn about diet and nutrition. Even when you know a lot of nutritional information, what works for some bodies is not necessarily what will work for others. And the needs for a growing body will change as that body matures and ages.

Now that you know a lot more about what you are eating, use what you've learned as a foundation to build on.

Try foods you haven't tried before.

Try different combinations.

Get creative and come up with your own recipes.

Find what you like that makes you feel full and makes you feel good afterward.

And if you have plenty to eat every day and plenty of choices, be thankful. You're lucky. Take advantage of it and enjoy what you are eating!